Health Technical Memorandum 2024

Validation and verification

Lifts

London: HMSO

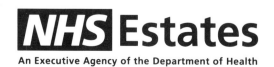

NHS Estates

An Executive Agency of the Department of Health

© Crown copyright 1995

Applications for reproduction should be made to HMSO Copyright Unit

First published 1995

ISBN 0 11 322208 4

HMSO
Standing order service

Placing a standing order with HMSO BOOKS enables a customer to receive future titles in this series automatically as published. This saves the time, trouble and expense of placing individual orders and avoids the problem of knowing when to do so. For details please write to HMSO BOOKS (PC 13A/1), Publications Centre, PO Box 276, London SW8 5DT quoting reference 14.02.017. The standing order service also enables customers to receive automatically as published all material of their choice which additionally saves extensive catalogue research. The scope and selectivity of the service has been extended by new techniques, and there are more than 3,500 classifications to choose from. A special leaflet describing the service in detail may be obtained on request.

About this publication

Health Technical Memoranda (HTMs) give comprehensive advice and guidance on the design, installation and operation of specialised building and engineering technology used in the delivery of healthcare.

They are applicable to new and existing sites, and are of use at various stages during the inception, design, construction, refurbishment and maintenance of a building.

Health Technical Memorandum 2024

HTM 2024 focuses on the:

    a. legal and mandatory requirements;

    b. design applications;

    c. commissioning;

    d. maintenance; and

    e. operation

of lifts in all types of healthcare premises.

It is published as four separate volumes each addressing a specialist discipline:

- **Management policy** – outlines the overall responsibility of chief executives and managers of healthcare premises, and details their legal and mandatory obligations in installing and operating a reliable, efficient and economic lift (vertical transportation) service. It summarises the technical aspects involved;

- **Design considerations** – details the requirements and considerations that apply to the design of lifts up to preparation stage of the contract document. Guidance is given on lift types and categories, capacities, planning new facilities, construction, electrical supplies and drives, safety features and hydraulic applications;

- this volume – **Validation and verification** – details the requirements for ensuring that manufactured equipment is formally tested and certified as to contract particulars, and manufactured to the highest level of quality assurance. The importance of commissioning is emphasised and the order of tests on site is listed;

- **Operational management** – provides information for those responsible for overseeing and operating day-to-day running and maintenance procedures. Coverage includes routine tests, planned preventive maintenance and troubleshooting.

Guidance in this Health Technical Memorandum is complemented by the library of National Health Service Model Engineering Specifications. Users of the guidance are advised to refer to the relevant specifications for "Lifts".

The contents of this Health Technical Memorandum in terms of management policy, operational policy and technical guidance are endorsed by:

a. the Welsh Office for the NHS in Wales;

b. the Health and Personal Social Services Management Executive in Northern Ireland;

c. the National Health Service in Scotland Management Executive.

Statutory guidance on electrical safety to meet the Electricity at Work Regulations 1989 is published in HTM 2020 – 'Electrical safety code for low voltage systems' and HTM 2021 – 'Electrical safety code for high voltage systems'.

Guidance on emergency electrical requirements is published in HTM 2011 – 'Emergency electrical services'. Guidance on electrical distribution is published in HTM 2007 – 'Electrical services: supply and distribution' and on reduction of electrical interference in HTM 2014 – 'Abatement of electrical interference'. Reference should also be made to HTM 2050 – 'Risk management in the NHS estate'.

References to legislation appearing in the main text of this guidance apply in England and Wales. Where references differ for Scotland and/or Northern Ireland, these are given as marginal notes. Where appropriate, marginal notes are also used to amplify the text.

Contents

1.0 Scope

General

Throughout this document, healthcare premises have also been referred to as hospitals. They will also include "social services premises" in Northern Ireland

Lifts in healthcare premises provide an essential service that may not always be fully appreciated by the users

1.1   Healthcare premises are dependent upon lifts to provide an efficient, fast and comfortable vertical transportation service for the movement of patients, staff, visitors, medical equipment and ancillary services items.

1.2   All lifts are subject to strict statutory regulations which cover operational safety to ensure that passengers can be fully confident that the lift service is safe to use.

1.3   The scope of this Health Technical Memorandum does not cover manual lifts, hoists, escalators and paternosters. Paternosters are considered too hazardous in a healthcare environment.

User considerations

1.4   The psychological aspects of lift design in terms of being user-friendly need to be addressed to allay anxieties and fears of users.

1.5   Travelling in a lift can be perceived as dangerous by persons of a nervous disposition, in several different ways, but mainly from the notion of being isolated in a sealed box inside a vertical well which extends from the lowest ground floor level to the top floor of the building.

1.6   A common claustrophobic fear is that of being trapped between floors without the means to communicate with persons outside to give warning of the predicament or to receive reassurance that assistance is at hand.

1.7   Physiological constraints affect the rates of acceleration and deceleration which the human body can comfortably withstand and in healthcare premises, the selection of operational lift speed is important to minimise any adverse effects on patients.

1.8   Psychological appreciations are more subtle and can be influenced by the lift finishes, decor, apparent reliability, frequency and transit time of the service.

2.0 Management responsibilities

2.1 It is incumbent on management to ensure that their lift installations comply with all the statutory regulations applicable to lifts on their premises. Other functional guidance in terms of standards and codes of practice should also be noted.

Statutory requirements

2.2 Safety regulations are as laid down in the:

a. Offices, Shops and Railway Premises (Hoists and Lifts) Regulations 1968;

Offices and Shop Premises (Hoists and Lifts) Regulations (Northern Ireland) 1969

b. Health and Safety at Work etc Act 1974;

Health and Safety at Work (Northern Ireland) Order 1978

c. Electricity at Work Regulations 1989;

Electricity at Work Regulations (Northern Ireland) 1991

d. Fire Precautions Act 1971 (as amended by the Fire Safety and Safety of Places of Sport Act 1987);

Fire Services (Northern Ireland) Order 1984 (as amended by the Fire Services (1984 Order) (Modifications) (Northern Ireland) 1993)

e. Factories Act 1961 (as amended);

Factories Act (Northern Ireland) 1965

f. Building Act 1984 and the Building Regulations 1991 (including Approved Documents);

Building Regulations (Northern Ireland) 1994
Building Standards (Scotland) Regulations 1990

g. Lifting Plant and Equipment (Record of Test and Examination etc) Regulations 1992;

Lifting Plant and Equipment (Record of Test and Examination etc) Regulations (Northern Ireland) 1993

h. Management of Health and Safety at Work Regulations 1992;

Management of Health and Safety at Work Regulations (Northern Ireland) 1992

j. Workplace (Health, Safety and Welfare) Regulations 1992;

Workplace (Health, Safety and Welfare) Regulations (Northern Ireland) 1993

k. Construction (Design and Management) Regulations 1994;

m. Reporting of Injuries, Diseases and Dangerous Occurrences Regulations 1985 (RIDDOR);

Reporting of Injuries, Diseases and Dangerous Occurrences Regulations (Northern Ireland) 1986

n. Electromagnetic Compatibility Regulations 1992, and the Electromagnetic Compatibility (Amendment) Regulations 1994;

p. Supply of Machinery (Safety) Regulations 1992.

Functional guidance

2.3   Guidance is as laid down in:

a.   British Standards and Codes of Practice;

b.   Health and Safety Executive Guidance;

c.   NHS Model Engineering Specifications – NHS Estates;

d.   Health Building Notes – NHS Estates;

e.   Technical Standards (Scotland);

f.   Health Technical Memoranda and Firecode – NHS Estates.

For further details on this guidance please refer to the references section.

2.4   The Offices, Shops and Railway Premises (Hoists and Lifts) Regulations 1968 require that a lift will function without injury or danger to the general public and passengers.

Safety applications

Competent person (lifts) – refer to Chapter 10 'Designated staff functions'

2.5   The Factories Act 1961 and the Offices, Shops and Railway Premises (Hoists and Lifts) Regulations 1968 require that every power-driven lift should be of good mechanical construction, sound material, adequate strength, properly maintained and thoroughly examined by a competent person (lifts) at least once in a period of six months, and that a report of the result of every such examination should be prepared on the prescribed form F2530 (previously F54) (see the 'Operational management' volume of this HTM), signed and dated by the person carrying out the examination.

2.6   The report should be retained and kept readily available for inspection for at least two years after the date of the lift examination.

2.7   The legal responsibility for ensuring that lifts are properly maintained rests with the management of the healthcare premises in which the lifts are installed.

2.8   At present, while there is no legal requirement for new lifts to be tested before being taken into service, it is strongly recommended that all lifts should be examined and tested in accordance with BS5655:Part 1:1986, by a competent person (lifts).

2.9   Fire regulations require that certain lift controls can be operated by the fire brigade so that firemen can take immediate control of the lift for safety and fire-fighting purposes.

2.10 At least one bed-lift in an acute hospital should be connected to the emergency electrical supply system in line with the guidance contained in HTM 2011 – 'Emergency electrical services'.

2.11 All passenger and bed/passenger lifts should be fitted with an emergency intercommunication point.

3.0 Functional overview

Types of lift

3.1   There are two main types of lift installed in healthcare premises; these are:

a. traction lifts;

b. hydraulic lifts.

Consideration should be given to the running (maintenance) costs incurred over the life span of the lift installation when comparisons are made between traction and hydraulic lifts.

Traction lifts

3.2   Traction lifts are most commonly used in high-rise buildings. They are rope-driven where the drive is by an electric variable speed motor, through a gearbox. The lift car travels vertically up and down the lift well between the lowest ground floor and the top floor. The lift car's weight is counterbalanced throughout its full travel.

3.3   Magnetic brake systems control the lift car movements between landing levels. In the event of an overtravel, the bottom of the lift well is cushioned by a buffer recoil mechanism. First and second overtravel limit switches ensure that there is adequate clearance at the top of the car for the safety of maintenance personnel.

3.4   The traction lift is versatile and can be designed to operate at very fast speeds, such as is required in high-rise buildings. Passenger lifts can routinely carry up to 21 passengers (1.6 tonnes) at speeds of 0.5 to 3.5 metres per second (100 to 700 ft/min), depending on travel and duty.

Hydraulic lifts

3.5   Hydraulic lifts are suitable for applications in low-rise buildings usually up to a maximum of four floors. They utilise less plantroom space and, in general, the overall capital cost is lower than for the traction lift.

3.6   The hydraulic lift is powered by oil-operated ram(s). For the direct acting type, the rams are located below or to the side of the lift car and for the indirect action type it is usual to have a driving mechanism with a side jack arrangement. The extended vertical length of the ram is physically limited and this in turn limits its suitability for low-rise buildings.

3.7   Hydraulic lifts generally operate at a slower speed in the raise direction than when travelling downwards. Lowering is by gravity and is speed controlled by restrictors in the hydraulic oil return path from the ram(s) to the hydraulic pump reservoir tank.

Categories of lift

3.8 Lifts are categorised according to their use. In healthcare premises they fall into one of the following categories:

a. **passenger lifts:** intended to carry standing and wheelchair-seated passengers. Typical carrying capacity varies from 600 to 1000 kg;

b. **bed/passenger lifts:** generally constructed to similar standards as passenger lifts but have a car of larger dimensions. This permits the carrying of a passenger (patient) on a bed or trolley together with the necessary staff and equipment. Typical carrying capacity varies from 1660 to 2500 kg;

c. **goods lifts:** typically carry up to 5 tonnes. Goods lifts that are also used to carry passengers should conform in all respects to the regulations governing the use of passenger lifts;

d. **service lifts:** service lifts are not designed to carry passengers. They are arranged to be called and despatched externally, normally by a call point adjacent to each level hatch or access door, and are generally used for small loads.

4.0 Testing and inspection criteria

4.1 Lifts in healthcare premises are subject to a statutory regime of inspection. Management should ensure that its operational procedures include the nomination of individuals to keep lifts in the required safe condition and to arrange for the mandatory inspections to be carried out at the prescribed intervals.

4.2 Every power-driven lift should be thoroughly examined at least once every six months (see paragraph 2.5). Lift examination should be supervised and performed only by an appointed competent person (lifts). It is therefore of the utmost importance that safety requirements are borne in mind at all times and that only approved and regulated procedures are applied.

4.3 Lifts are subject to the Electricity at Work Regulations 1989. Compliance is obtained by ensuring that only authorised personnel have access to electrical equipment and supplies. Electrical wiring and circuits in lift cars must be securely enclosed to prevent unauthorised access. Similarly, lift motor rooms and hydraulic machine rooms should be kept locked and the procedures of HTM 2020 – 'Electrical safety code for low voltage systems' strictly applied.

4.4 Healthcare premises are subject to the requirements of the Health and Safety at Work etc Act 1974. The Health and Safety guidance note PM7 recommends that the inspection standards contained in the Factories Act 1961 and the Offices, Shops and Railway Premises (Hoists and Lifts) Regulations 1968 be applied in other work places, including healthcare premises. Health and Safety Executive HM Factory Inspectorate Form F2530 (previously F54) has to be completed for any lift installations to which these Acts apply.

4.5 Insurance companies will only provide cover for lifts if the legal inspection requirements have been met. It is customary for their inspectors to carry out the statutory examination of lifts which they insure. It should be noted that insurance inspection reports refer to the condition of the lift at the time of inspection. Local management is responsible for ensuring that a satisfactory standard is maintained.

4.6 The purpose of thorough examination and testing is to ascertain whether the lift installation may continue to remain safely in service.

5.0 Commissioning principles

5.1 Commissioning is all the activities that are undertaken prior to the lift going into service which ensure that the lift complies with the specified requirements and that optimum performance is achieved.

5.2 Lift manufacturers have a responsibility to ensure that the delivered goods are in accordance with the contract specification.

5.3 Differences may occur, however, as a result of a breakdown in communication at one of the stages between the offer and the commissioning stage.

5.4 The manufacture of a lift, from specification to commissioning, can involve several parties, often on an international scale.

5.5 At various stages of the manufacturing process, the contract specification may be broken down into segments and transposed into "internal instruction", or even translated into foreign languages to suit the manufacturer's sources. Some of the details of the specification may be lost during this process and result in a "standard product" being offered.

5.6 Installation and lift manufacturer's commissioning staff may not be in possession of the contract specification for reference. They will therefore normally install and commission the delivered equipment in accordance with their standard procedures.

5.7 Healthcare premises management may wish to supplement these checks by having inspection undertaken by their own personnel or by a third party if in-house lift expertise is not available. Such third parties may be insurance companies or consultancies who specialise in lift engineering. However, insurance companies are primarily involved in ensuring a safe installation and may not be able to offer the depth of expertise to advise on the overall commissioning of complex controls and drive systems.

5.8 Within the framework of the Health and Safety at Work etc Act 1974, a supplier has the duty to ensure that the equipment is suitable and "safe" for the stated intended purpose.

6.0 Validation of tender/specification

6.1 The required inspection, testing and commissioning should be clearly stated in the contract specification so that adequate provisions are incorporated into the offer.

6.2 As a prerequisite to commissioning, all relevant contract documents including contract specifications, detailed drawings and details of all variations agreed or instructed since the original order was placed, should be made available.

6.3 The documentation supplied by the lift manufacturer should be checked for compliance with the contract specification (and subsequent variations). All errors, deviations and omissions should be notified in writing to the manufacturer via the contractual route.

6.4 Any error corrected at this stage will prevent costly site changes and delays in completion.

6.5 This validation stage may reveal oversights of detail or the inclusion of the lift maker's variations to match their standard production item.

6.6 The failure to identify obscure omissions or variations at this validation stage will not relieve the lift manufacturer from his contractual obligations.

6.7 Once the contract is in place and the supply of the lift is in progress, a programme of checks should be undertaken as defined in the contract specification. Typically the programme of checks would comprise the following:

   a. off site: checks during manufacture for major pieces of equipment;

   b. on site: during installation;

   c. on site: upon completion;

   d. on site: when in service.

7.0 Checks during manufacture

7.1 A lift installation will invariably comprise a combination of the lift manufacturer's own equipment and bought-in components.

7.2 Reputable lift manufacturers will ensure compliance with the specified requirements by following quality systems such as BS EN 5750 ISO 9000 Quality Assurance. Quality systems would include batch testing of components, checking of machining, fabrication, packaging, etc and the testing of the assembled sub-component or unit.

7.3 These systems may already be in place but may be supplemented by specific requirements to suit a particular application.

It is recommended that type test certificates, from an approved test house, are called for by the client in his/her tender invitation and provided by the contractor in his/her submission. This works test certificate should be available on site prior to the commencement of "site commissioning"

7.4 Each major item of equipment should have been type tested. It is recommended that works tests should be completed on these items for which a prototype "test certificate" is issued. This includes all equipment that has been manufactured to specific British or international standards.

7.5 Works tests are also recommended where the equipment being produced is unique in any way, or is of such complexity that modification must take place before delivery.

7.6 These tests may include, for example, works testing and simulation of control panels where unique functions have been incorporated, or where the first unit of a large order is produced for "prototype" approval.

8.0 Site checks during installation

8.1   Prior to the delivery of equipment to site, the lift manufacturer should carry out checks on the lift well to ensure that the dimensions, plumbness, location of fixings, etc comply with builder's agreed work drawings.

8.2   Lifts are generally supplied to the site as consignments of components for assembly in the lift well. Not all of the components would have been procured from a single source and they might be delivered at different times to suit the stages of installation.

8.3   The lift equipment may comprise pre-assembled components delivered as larger units. This equipment may require further adjustment and re-alignment when installed, but should have been protected from damage during transportation and storage by correct packaging and handling.

8.4   The lift manufacturer should maintain a "sight quality plan" which will list all checks together with relevant documentation including drawings, quantities, location, manufacturer's setting-up data and certificates.

8.5   The "sight quality plan" should include such information as guide rail plumbing charts which may be examined to verify correct installation parameters.

8.6   It should be remembered that the lift installation process is a constant progression up to the final commissioning stage. Management's observation should be directed at identifying unacceptable standards of completed work, and equipment which does not comply with the contract specification, has been damaged or is inadequately protected in site storage.

When the installation has reached practical completion in accordance with the contract, a take-over certificate should be issued certifying the date on which the installation was taken over and the commencement of the maintenance/defects liability period

9.0 Checks upon completion – commissioning

9.1 BS5655: Part 10: 1986 recommends a standard form for reporting lift tests. However, this requires information to be recorded in a yes/no or pass/fail format often without finite values recorded.

Wiring diagrams, instruction manuals, etc should be made available, preferably at the time of commissioning but no later than at hand-over. Refer to HTM 2007 for details of testing electrical services

9.2 In healthcare premises, it is important that all the records of the lifts installed are documented. This will enable comparisons to be made between the original commissioning figures and any subsequent routine test results. These comparisons will identify any deterioration or excessive variations beyond the commissioning parameters.

The samples referred to cover both mechanical and electrical tests

9.3 Guidance sample sheets, based on a variation of BS5655: Part 10: 1986 test formats, are listed in Appendices 1 and 2. They depict typical formats that can be used as the basis of a commissioning report for traction and hydraulic lifts in healthcare premises.

10.0 Designated staff functions

10.1 Only trained authorised and competent persons (lifts) should be appointed by management to control the operation and maintenance of lifts.

10.2 Management: the owner, occupier, employer, general manager, chief executive or other person who is accountable for the premises and is responsible for issuing or implementing a general policy statement under the Health and Safety at Work etc (HSW) Act 1974.

10.3 Designated person (electrical): an individual who has overall authority and responsibility for the premises containing the electrical supply and distribution system within the premises and has a duty under the HSW Act 1974 to prepare and issue a general policy statement on health and safety at work, including the organisation and arrangements for carrying out that policy. This person should not be the authorising engineer.

10.4 Designated person (lifts): an individual who has been nominated by management to ensure that lift operations are kept to a satisfactory standard including mandatory examinations, record keeping and emergency procedures.

10.5 Duty holder: a person on whom the Electricity at Work Regulations 1989 impose a duty in connection with safety.

10.6 Competent person (lifts): a person with adequate training, both theoretical and practical, and with experience of the equipment (lift installation) under examination to enable a true assessment of its continued safe operation to be made and who is supported within an appropriate organisation.

This definition of competent person (lifts) is synonymous with the definition of authorised person as defined in BS7255: 1989

10.7 Employer: any person or body who:

a. employs one or more individuals under a contract of employment or apprenticeship;

b. provides training under the schemes to which the Health and Safety (Training for Employment) Regulations 1990 (SI 1380: 1990) apply.

Northern Ireland: Health and Safety (Training for Employment) Regulations 1994 (SI 1: 1994)

10.8 Authorising engineer (high voltage): a chartered electrical engineer with appropriate experience and possessing the necessary degree of independence from local management who is appointed in writing by management to implement, administer and monitor the safety arrangements for the high voltage electrical supply and distribution systems of that organisation to ensure compliance with the Electricity at Work Regulations 1989 and to assess the suitability and appointment of candidates in writing to be authorised persons (see HTM 2021 – 'Electrical safety code for high voltage systems').

10.9 Authorising engineer (low voltage): a chartered engineer or incorporated electrical engineer with appropriate experience and possessing the necessary degree of independence from local management who is appointed in writing by management to implement, administer and monitor the safety arrangements for the low voltage electrical supply and distribution systems of that organisation to ensure compliance with the Electricity at Work Regulations 1989 and to assess the suitability and appointment of candidates in writing to be authorised persons (see HTM 2020 – 'Electrical safety code for low voltage systems').

10.10 Authorised person (electrical): an individual possessing adequate technical knowledge and having received appropriate training, appointed in writing by the authorising engineer to be responsible for the practical implementation and operation of management's safety policy and procedures on defined electrical systems (see HTM 2021 and HTM 2020).

10.11 Competent person (electrical): an individual who, in the opinion of an authorised person, has sufficient technical knowledge and experience to prevent danger while carrying out work on defined electrical systems (see HTM 2021 and HTM 2020).

11.0 Definitions

11.1 Department: an abbreviation of the generic term "UK Health Departments" (the Department of Health, the Scottish Office, the Welsh Office and the Department of Health and Social Services Northern Ireland).

11.2 Lift: an appliance for transporting persons or goods between two or more levels by means of a guided car moving in a substantially vertical direction and travelling in the same path in both upward and downward directions (BS).

11.3 Traction lift: a lift whose lifting ropes are driven by friction in the grooves of the driving sheave of the machine (BS).

11.4 Hydraulic lift: a lift in which the lifting power is derived from an electrically-driven pump, transmitting hydraulic fluid to a jack, acting directly or indirectly on the car (BS).

11.5 System: a system in which all the electrical equipment is, or may be, electrically connected to a common source of electrical energy, including such source and such equipment.

11.6 Injury: death or personal injury from electrical or mechanical failures.

11.7 Danger: a risk of injury.

11.8 Essential circuits: circuits forming part of the essential services electrical supply so arranged that they can be supplied separately from the remainder of the electrical installation.

11.9 Emergency supply: any form of electrical supply which is intended to be available in the event of a failure in the normal supply.

11.10 Essential service electrical supply: the supply from an engine-driven a.c. emergency generator which is arranged to come into operation in the event of a failure of the normal supply and provide sufficient electrical energy to ensure that all basic functions of the healthcare premises are maintained in service.

11.11 Electrical equipment: includes anything used, intended to be used or installed for use to generate, provide, transmit, transform, conduct, distribute, control, measure or use electrical energy.

11.12 High voltage (HV): the existence of a potential difference (rms value for a.c.) normally exceeding 1000 volts a.c. between circuit conductors or 600 volts between circuit conductors and earth.

11.13 Low voltage (LV): the existence of a potential difference (rms value for a.c.) not exceeding 1000 volts a.c. or 1500 volts d.c. between circuit conductors or 600 volts a.c. or 900 volts d.c. between circuit conductors and earth.

Appendix 1

Sample certificate of test and examination for electrical traction passenger and goods lifts

---

Certificate of test and examination for electric traction passenger and goods lifts

Notes for the completion of this certificate

NOTE 1.   The references quoted below in association with BS part number refer to clauses, figures, tables or appendices to that Part 1 of BS5655. Other clause numbers relate to this Part of BS5655.

NOTE 2.   Statements and replies to all relevant questions should be annotated in the appropriate boxes. Where multiple questions are posed, only one of the alternative boxes should be ticked.

1.1   Description of installation

Location :

Vendor :

Length of travel :   m

No. of levels served :

Vendor's identification No. :

No. of entrances served :   front

Hospital Lift Asset No./Hospital I.D. No.

rear

side

Power supply at time of test :

Rated load :   kg   persons

Rated speed :   m/s

	specified	actual	
			Voltage
			Phase
			Hz
			Wire
			Fuse Type
			Fuse Rating

Machine room location :

permanent

temporary

Machine room temperature at the start of the dynamic tests :   °C

Earth loop impedance N/A

Is a power retest required?

Yes   No

State Reason :

Key Wiring Diag. Nos :

17

1.2 Static examination, mechanical

1.2.1 Suspension

(a) State :

	specified	actual
(1) Number		
(2) Nominal diameter		
(3) Lay & Construction		

	Car	Counterweight
(b) Type of rope anchorages		
(c) If rope grips are used : (1) State the number fitted per rope termination		MIN FOUR Yes ☐
(2) Are grips fitted correctly ?		Yes ☐ No ☐
(d) If socket anchorages are used, state type :		
(e) If any other type of anchorage is used, describe it :		

(f) Is the rope test certificate available
and in order ?   Yes ☐   No ☐

(g) Are the rope anchorages in accordance
with 9.2.3. of Part 2 ?   Yes ☐   No ☐

(h) If eyebolts are used do they comply
with Part 8 ?   Yes ☐   No ☐

(i) Is rope compensation fitted ?   Yes ☐   No ☐

(j) State type, mass/metre, and construction   ☐

(k) Is slack compensating rope switch fitted ?   Yes ☐   No ☐

1.2.2 Safety gear

(a) Has the safety gear been certified as complying
with F.3 and in accordance with F.3.5. of Part 1 ?   Yes ☐   No ☐

(b) If foregoing answer is 'Yes' is the data plate fitted
and in accordance with 15.14 of Part 1 ?   Yes ☐   No ☐

(c) Is the safety gear sealed ?   Instantaneous   N/A ☐   Yes ☐   No ☐

Progressive   N/A ☐   Yes ☐   No ☐

1.2.3 Car

(a)   State the internal width (wall to wall)
(without finishes) :

(b)   State the internal depth (front return to rear wall or
front return to rear return) (without finishes) :

(c)   Does the available internal floor area, related to
rated load and maximum number of passengers, comply   Yes   No
with 8.2 of Part 1 ?

1.2.4   Energy accumulation buffers (e.g. spring)   N/A ☐

   (a)   If fitted, do buffers comply to 10.4.1. of Part 1 ?   Yes ☐   No ☐

Note: It is recommended that buffers should have been identified with their spring rate maximum load and maker's name.

	CAR	COUNTERWEIGHT
State quantity	Qty :	Qty :
State type if other than spring	Type :	Type :

1.2.5   Energy dissipation buffers (e.g. oil)   N/A ☐

   (a)   Are they correctly filled and not leaking ?   Yes ☐   No ☐

   (b)   Is the stroke of each buffer in accordance with 10.4.3 of Part 1 ?   Yes ☐   No ☐

1.2.6   Hydraulic fluid (see BS 4231)

Maker : ☐   Type : ☐   Viscosity grade : ☐

1.2.7   Overspeed governor

   (a)   State type of Overspeed governor   e.g. Clamp/traction   ☐

   (b)   Has the governor been certified as complying with F.4 and as being in accordance with F4.3. of Part 1 ?   Yes ☐   No ☐

   (c)   Is the data plate in accordance with 15.6 of Part 1 ?   Yes ☐   No ☐

   (d)   Is the governor sealed ?   Yes ☐   No ☐

1.2.8   Overspeed governor rope

   (a)   Is the nominal diameter of rope appropriate ?   Yes ☐   No ☐

	specified	actual
(b) State size :		
(c) Construction :		

1.2.9   Landing doors and surrounds

(a)   Does the contract require that the landing doors and
surrounds satisfy appropriate fire rating requirements ?   Yes   ☐

If so, what is the fire rating requirement ?   ☐ h

(b)   If the answer to (a) is Yes, is the test certificate available
and in order ?   Yes   ☐   No   ☐

(c)   If so, and doors are manually operated, is the means of
fire protection a fusible link ?   Yes   ☐   No   ☐

If the answer is 'No', describe method used :   ☐

(d)   Are the fire rated elements of the door assembly
correctly fitted ?   Yes   ☐   No   ☐

1.2.10   Door locks

(a)   Have the door locks been certified
as complying with F.1.4 of Part 2 ?   Yes   ☐   No   ☐

If 'Yes' does the data plate comply with
15.13 of Part 2 ?   Yes   ☐   No   ☐

1.3   Static examination, electrical

1.3.1   Insulation resistance to earth (see clause 5)

(a)   Lift Motor   ☐ MΩ   Measured at 1000V D.C.

(b)   M-G Set (if fitted)   motor   ☐ MΩ   generator   ☐ MΩ

(c)   Power System   ☐ MΩ   Measured at 1000V D.C.

(d)   Safety Circuit   ☐ MΩ   Measured at 500V D.C.

1.3.2   Earthing

(a)   Is the maximum continuity resistance to earth
less than 0.5Ω ?   Yes   ☐   No   ☐

(b)   Is the car connected to controller earthing terminal
by a separate conductor no smaller than 0.75 mm² ?   Yes   ☐   No   ☐

(c)   Does the earth loop impedance comply with fuse
rating ?   Yes   ☐   No   ☐   reading ☐

1.3.3 Protection of conductors

(a) Is the fixed wiring in conduit (or trunking)
or fittings which ensure equivalent protection
throughout ?

Yes ☐   No ☐

or

(b) If 'No' do cables comply with 13.5.1.2.
of Part 1 ?

N/A ☐   Yes ☐   No ☐

1.3.4 Phase failure device

Does the phase reversal and phase failure
protection operate correctly ?

Yes ☐   No ☐

1.3.5 Electrical conductors

Do the electrical conductors, including travelling
cables, comply with 13.5.1 Part 1 ?

Yes ☐   No ☐

1.4.1 Safety contacts/circuits

(a) Have the contacts at each landing entrance been proved so that when broken there is no movement of the car ? Yes ☐ No ☐

(b) Have the car door/gate contacts been proved so that when open circuited there is no car movement outside the unlocking zone ? Yes ☐ No ☐

(c) Have the stopping devices on car top and in the pulley room and pit been proved so that when open circuited no movement of the car occurs ? Yes ☐ No ☐

(d) Have all other switches/contacts in safety circuits been proved so that when open circuited no movement of the car occurs ? Yes ☐ No ☐

(e) Does the earthing of the most remote contact (lock or push button) operate a fuse or trip a circuit breaker without delay ? Yes ☐ No ☐

(f) Have the mechanical locks at each landing entrance been provided for positive locking ? Yes ☐ No ☐

(g) If separate terminal stopping switches are fitted, do they operate satisfactorily ? N/A ☐ Yes ☐ No ☐

(h) Do the final limit switches operate satisfactorily ? Yes ☐ No ☐

(i) Final limit switch settings. State distance to operate beyond finished floor level. specified / actual Top ☐ ☐ Bottom ☐ ☐

1.4.2 Car top control station (with a load of 75 Kg)

(a) Speed up : ☐ m/s   (b) Speed down : ☐ m/s

(b) Does the design and operation of car top station comply with clause 14.2.1.3 of Part 1? Yes ☐ No ☐

(c) Is a door open/close switch fitted ? Yes ☐ No ☐

(d) On open through cars is there a stop push within 1m of the rear entrance ? Yes ☐ No ☐

1.4.3 Clearances and runbys

(a) Will the car and counterweight clear all obstacles when driven at slow speed :

    (1) With the car and rated load on to and fully compressing the car buffers ?   Yes ☐ No ☐

    (2) With the counterweight compressing its buffers (car full) ?   Yes ☐ No ☐

(b) What is the distance to the first striking point above the car with the counterweight on the compressed buffer ?   [_____] mm

Does this comply with 5.7.1.1 of Part 1 ?   Yes ☐ No ☐

(c) What is the estimated distance to the first striking point above the counterweight with the car on compressed buffer ?

    Is this at least 300 mm ?   Yes ☐ No ☐

(d) With the car on its fully compressed buffers, is there sufficient space to accommodate the rectangular block specified in 5.7.3.3 of Part 1 and at least 0.5 m between the bottom part of the pit and the lowest part of the car ?   Yes ☐ No ☐

    State the dimension   [_____] mm

Note. The clear distance between the bottom of the pit and the lowest part of the guide shoes or safety gear block, or toe guards or parts of vertical sliding doors, should be at least 0.1 m.

1.4.4 Entrance clearances

(a) Is the horizontal distance between the sill of the car and the sill of all landing doors 35 mm or less ?
For each set of doors   Yes ☐ No ☐

(b) Is the running clearance between door panels, and between panels and uprights, lintels or sills 6 mm or less ?   Yes ☐ No ☐

(c) Has it been established that no recess or projection on the face of the sliding door panels exceeds 3 mm ?   Yes ☐ No ☐

(d) Is the distance between the inner surface of the well and the sill and framework of the car entrance or door <= 0.15 m or 0.2 m if over a height not exceeding 0.5 m (see 5.4.3.2 of Part 2) ?   Yes ☐ No ☐

(e) If the answer to (d) is 'No', is the car door mechanically locked when away from the unlocking zone in accordance with 8.11.1 of Part 2 ?   Yes ☐ No ☐

1.4.5 Door tests

NOTE : Where appropriate the following tests should be carried out with car and landing doors coupled

(a) How are the doors operated ? manually ☐ if so, answer f,h,i,j,k,l

powered ☐ if so, answer all except l

(b) Is the measured maximum force to prevent closing, at Yes ☐ No ☐
the mid-point of travel, 150 N or less ?

State the figure recorded : ☐ N

1.4.5 Door tests (continued)

(c) Is the measured kinetic energy 10 J or less ?　　Yes [ ]　No [ ]

State the figure recorded :　[ ]

(d) Do all the protective devices reverse the doors in accordance with 7.5.2.1.1. of Part 2 ? Includes all mechanical or electrical devices supplied.　　Yes [ ]　No [ ]

(e) If the protective device is made inoperative :

(1) Do the doors remain open ?　　Yes [ ]　No [ ]

(2) Do the doors close with a kinetic energy not exceeding 4 J ?　N/A [ ]　Yes [ ]　No [ ]

(f) Is the unlocking zone less than 0.2 m above and below landing levels (or 0.35 m in the case of simultaneously operated car and landing doors) ? Check length of retiring ramp and position of lock roller.　　Yes [ ]　No [ ]

(g) Do the landing doors have an automatic self-closing mechanism ?　　Yes [ ]　No [ ]

(h) Is each set of the landing doors capable of being unlocked from the outside with an emergency key ?　　Yes [ ]　No [ ]

If not, why ?　[ ]

(i) Does the door motor protection system function correctly ?　　Yes [ ]　No [ ]

Does the retiring actuator protection system function correctly ?　N/A [ ]　Yes [ ]　No [ ]

(j) Form of electrical protection provided for the door motor

D.C. circuit breaker	[ ]	Timing relay	[ ]
Three phase circuit breaker	[ ]	Thermistors	[ ]
Overloads in each phase	[ ]	Other (state)	Fuses

Form of electrical protection provided for the retiring actuator

D.C. circuit breaker	[ ]	Timing relay	[ ]
Three phase circuit breaker	[ ]	Thermistors	[ ]
Overloads in each phase	[ ]	Other (state)	Fuses

State the relevant characteristics :　CCT (swing) ODT/CDT (powered)

Time to operate [ ] s

Run current [ ] A

(k) Can the car doors be manually opened within the unlocking zone with a force of less than 300 N with the power off ?　　Yes [ ]　No [ ]

(l) Does "car here" indicator comply with 7.6.2 of Part 2 for manual doors ?　N/A [ ]

1.5 Measurements of the electrical system

(a) State power system

(b) Provide details of motor as on motor plate

    (1) Maker

    (2) Serial No.

    (3) Type

    (4) Power rating   kW

    (5) Current rating   A

    (6) Speed   rpm

    (7) Class of insulation

    (8) Duty Rating

(c) Measure the following operational data when the car is at the mid point of travel :

High speed operation									
Car loading condition		Lift motor speed (see note 3)	Lift speed (see note 3)	Lift motor input (see note 1)			System input (see note 2)			Levelling deviation (+ or −) (see note 4)
				RUN		START	RUN		START	
		r.p.m.	m/s	V	A	A	V	A	A	mm
Empty	Up									
	Down									
Balanced	Up									
	Down									
Rated	Up									
	Down									
110%	Up									
	Down									

Note 1 Take the motor current readings on conductors adjacent to motor terminals with motor running steadily.
Note 2 Energy convertor or equivalent e.g. VVVF. Measure the system input from the mains supply.
Note 3 Complete either column 2 or 3 in its entirety & only the rated up reading for the alternative column.
Note 4 State the maximum deviation in the box & identify which floor.

1.5 Electrical systems (continued)

Low speed operation (if applicable)									
Car loading condition		Lift motor speed (see note 3)	Lift speed (see note 3)	Lift motor input (see note 1)			System input (see note 2)			Levelling deviation (+ or −) (see note 4)
				RUN		START	RUN		START	
		r.p.m.	m/s	V	A	A	V	A	A	mm
Empty	Up									
	Down									
Balanced	Up									
	Down									
Rated	Up									
	Down									
110%	Up									
	Down									

Note 1 Take the motor current readings on conductors adjacent to motor terminals with motor running steadily.
Note 2 Energy convertor or equivalent e.g. VVVF. Measure the system input from the mains supply.
Note 3 Complete either column 2 or 3 in its entirety & only the rated up reading for the alternative column.
Note 4 State the maximum deviation in the box & identify which floor.

(d)   Quote type of, and the following data on, the associated energy convertors (drive) name plate :

(1) Type

(2) Manufacturer

(3) Serial Number

(4) Input   kW   A   V

(5) Output   kW   A   V

1.6.1 Motor main windings over current protective devices

(a) Measure and record the follwing (as appropriate) :

Type of device	Manual reset		Automatic reset		Time to operate		Trip current	
Three phase circuit breaker								
Overloads in each phase								
Timing relay (TR1)								
Thermistor (TCU)								
Other : name type								

(b) Have you found these to operate satisfactorily ?   Yes ☐   No ☐

1.6.2 Slow speed windings

Type of device	Manual reset		Automatic reset		Time to operate		Trip current	
Three phase circuit breaker								
Overloads in each phase								
Timing relay (TR1)								
Thermistor (TCU)								
Other : name type								

Have you found these to operate satisfactorily ?   Yes ☐   No ☐

1.6.3 Convertor input

Type of device	Manual reset		Automatic reset		Time to operate		Trip current	
Three phase circuit breaker								
Overloads in each phase								
Timing relay (TR1)								
Thermistor (TCU)								
Other : name type								

Have you found these to operate satisfactorily ?   Yes ☐   No ☐

1.7 Overspeed governor tests

1.7.1 Car overspeed governor test   Complete the following :

Governor type :

Serial No. :

Device	Tripping speed		Does it operate effectively?	
	Marked	Measured (car down)	Yes	No
Electrical		m/s		
Mechanical	m/s	m/s		

1.7.2 Counterweight overspeed governor test   Complete the following :   N/A

Governor type :

Serial No. :

Device	Tripping speed		Does it operate effectively?	
	Marked	Measured (car down)	Yes	No
Electrical		m/s		
Mechanical	m/s	m/s		

State how the governors were tested on site

1.8 Car safety gear test

(a) To carry out the safety gear tests, the test load must be uniformly distributed in the car. The safety gear switch, overspeed governor switch, buffer switch or any other electrical devices that may cause the lift to stop by electrical means must be temporarily shorted-out.

N/A ☐

The tests must be conducted with the car descending, wth the brake open and the machine continuing to run at contract speed until the ropes slip on the sheave.

1.8.1 Progressive safety gear (Including type tested safety gears)

(a) Is the safety gear sealed ? Yes ☐ No ☐

(b) Does the stopping device operate correctly ? Yes ☐ No ☐

(c) For progressive safety gear state slide distance : ☐ mm

(d) Is the floor horizontal or sloping less than 5% (1 in 11) ? Yes ☐ No ☐

1.8.2 Instantaneous safety gear

(a) Is the safety gear sealed ? Yes ☐ No ☐

(b) Does the safety gear operate satisfactorily ? Yes ☐ No ☐

1.9 Counterweight safety gear

N/A ☐

(a) Counterweight safety gear : Yes ☐ No ☐

Test load = empty car

Test speed = car up rated speed

(b) For progressive safety gear state slide distance : ☐ m

(c) Does this value fall within those given in appendix ? Yes ☐ No ☐

1.10 Reduced stroke buffering

N/A ☐

Does the terminal speed reduction system ensure that the buffer impact speed is appropriate to the stroke of the buffer (see 10.4.3.2 of Part 1) ?   Yes ☐   No ☐

1.11 Buffers

1.11.1 Energy dissipation type (e.g. oil)

N/A ☐

(a) For car buffers, when the car was brought into contact with the buffers at the rated load, at rated speed or at a speed for which the stroke of the buffers has been calculated, was operation satisfactory ?   Yes ☐   No ☐

(b) For counterweight buffers, when the counterweight was brought into contact with the buffer with the car empty at rated speed, or at a speed for which the stroke of the buffer has been calculated, was the operation satisfactory ?   Yes ☐   No ☐

(c) Do the buffers recover automatically after operation ?   Yes ☐   No ☐

or

1.11.2 Energy accumulation buffers (e.g. spring)

N/A ☐

NOTE : If answer to 2.4. (a) is ''Yes'' no test required.

1.12 Traction checks

(a) Does the car stop under emergency conditions,

    (1) with the car empty when travelling upwards at rated speed ?   Yes ☐   No ☐

    (2) with the rated load plus 25% when travelling downwards in the lower part of the well at rated speed ?   Yes ☐   No ☐

(b) With the counterweight resting on its compressed buffer, is it impossible for the empty car to be raised under power ?   Yes ☐   No ☐

(c) From the measurements in 1.5 is the balance satisfactory ?   Yes ☐   No ☐

    State the percentage balance   Design ☐

    Actual ☐

(d) Does the lift stop within + or – 5 mm and remain within that tolerance during loading and unloading of single piece heavy items of not more than 25% rated load ?   Yes ☐   No ☐

1.13 Duty cycle test

(a) Does the lift operate satisfactorily for a period of at least 0.5 hours when running with rated load, full travel and intermediate stops at a rate of starts at least equal to the number of starts recommended in Part 6 ?   Yes ☐   No ☐

(b) If answer is "No" state reasons :

NOTE : It may be necessary to reduce door open timing to achieve the required number of starts per hour

1.14 General

(a) Is the maximum load indicated in the car (e.g. number of persons, kg and identification no.) and does it comply with 15.2.1 of Part 2 ?   Yes ☐   No ☐

(b) Does the fire fighting control system comply with the recommendations given in BS 5588 : Part 5 ?   N/A ☐   Yes ☐   No ☐

(c) Does the disabled evacuation system comply with the recommendations given in BS 5588 : Part 5 ?   N/A ☐   Yes ☐   No ☐

(d) Are the emergency instructions displayed in the machine room ?   Yes ☐   No ☐

(e) Does the emergency operation system(s) function correctly in accordance with 12.5 of Part 1 ?   Yes ☐   No ☐

If 'Yes', to whom has it been demonstrated ?

Name :

Organisation :

(f) Is the machine room artificial lighting adequate for maintenance purposes ?   Yes ☐   No ☐

(g) Does the artificial lighting in the well comply with 5.9. of Part 2 ?   Yes ☐   No ☐

(h) Are the machine room conditions satisfactory ?   Yes ☐   No ☐

If the answer is 'No', state reasons :

(i) Is the machine room adequately ventilated ?   Yes ☐   No ☐

(j) State the machine room temperature at the end of tests :

Is the temperature rise acceptable ?   Yes ☐   No ☐

(k) Are the machine room doors or trap doors fitted with a suitable lock complying with 6.3.3.3. of Part 2 ?   Yes ☐   No ☐

(l) What are the means of emergency communication for passengers in the lift car ?

Do they work ?   Yes ☐   No ☐

(m) Does the emergency lighting of the car stay illuminated for one hour ?   Yes ☐   No ☐

(n) Are there safe means of access to all items of equipment in accordance with Part 1 ?   Yes ☐   No ☐

If the answer is 'No', state reasons :

(o) Are the safety notices/instructions specified in clause 15 of Part 1 and recommended in Part 6 correctly displayed ?   Yes ☐   No ☐

(p) Has a car apron been fitted ?   Yes ☐   No ☐

(q) Has a counterweight screen been fitted ?   Yes ☐   No ☐

(r) If reduced headroom is applicable, are notices to this effect displayed in the pit and machine room ?   N/A ☐   Yes ☐   No ☐

1.15 Conclusions

(a) Is the lift installation complete and ready to be put into service ?   Yes ☐   No ☐

Note : Some items requiring attention may not be part of the contract for the lift but part of the installation and the responsibility of others. A list of inclusions and exclusions is given in Part 6

(b) If the answer to (a) is 'No', provide details in space below :

1.16 Declaration

I/We certify that on ☐ the equipment was thoroughly examined and found to be free from obvious defects and to comply with British Standard BS 5655 : Part 2, subject to any statement in 2.1.4 (b) above and that the foregoing is a correct report of the result.

Signature (s) :

Name and address of public service, association, company, firm or person making the examination :

Position in above organisation of the person who conducted the examination :

or

Qualifications of examiner, if working on his own account :

Appendix 2

Sample certificate of test and examination for hydraulic passenger and goods lifts

---

Certificate of test and examination for hydraulic passenger and goods lifts

---

Notes for the completion of this certificate

NOTE 1. The references quoted below in association with BS part number refer to clauses, figures, tables or appendices to that Part of BS 5655. Other clause numbers relate to this Part of BS 5655.

NOTE 2. Statements and replies to all relevant questions should be annotated in the appropriate boxes. Where multiple questions are posed, only one of the alternative boxes should be ticked.

2.1 Description of installation

Location :

Vendor :

Length of travel :   m

No. of levels served :

No. of entrances served :   front

                                   rear

                                   side

Vendor's identification No. :

Hospital Lift Asset No./Hospital I.D. No.

Power supply at time of test :

	specified	actual	
			Voltage
			Phase
			Hz
			Wire
			Fuse Type
			Fuse Rating

Rated load :   kg   persons

Rated speed up :   m/s

Rated speed down :   m/s

permanent

temporary

Earth loop impedance N/A

Machine room location :

Machine room temperature at the start of the dynamic tests :   °C

Is a power retest required ?

Yes   No

Number of rams :

Ram action :   direct acting   indirect acting

Type of ram :   single   telescopic

Ram dia(s) :

Quantity hyd hoses :   Dia :

Year of manufacture

State reason :

Key Wiring Diag. Nos :

2.2   Static examination, mechanical

2.2.1 Suspension

(a) If a direct acting lift :   N/A   ☐

(1) Is it fitted with a governor-operated safety gear ?   Yes ☐   No ☐

(2) Is it fitted with a rupture valve ?   Yes ☐   No ☐

(3) Is it fitted with a restrictor ?   Yes ☐   No ☐

---

or

(b) If an indirect acting lift :   N/A   ☐

(1) Is it fitted with a governor-operated safety gear ?   Yes ☐   No ☐

(2) Is it fitted with a safety-rope-operated safety
     gear and rupture valve ?   Yes ☐   No ☐

(3) Is it fitted with a safety-rope-operated safety
     gear and restrictor ?   Yes ☐   No ☐

2.2.1.1 Suspension ropes :

(a) State :

	specified	actual
(1) Number	☐	☐
(2) Nominal diameter	☐	☐
(3) Lay & construction	☐	☐

	Car	Pit Anchorage
(b) Type of rope anchorages * delete as appropriate	Ferrule secured eye with * eyebolt/*25 mm pin	Eyebolt, thimble & rope grips
(c) If rope grips are used : (1) State the number fitted per rope termination	N/A	FOUR Yes ☐
(2) Are grips fitted correctly ?	N/A	Yes ☐ No ☐
(d) If socket anchorages are used, state type :	N/A	N/A
(e) If any other type of anchorage is used, describe it :	N/A	

(f) Is the rope test certificate available
     and in order ?   Yes ☐   No ☐

(g) Are the rope anchorages in accordance
     with 9.2.3. of Part 2 ?   Yes ☐   No ☐

(h) If eyebolts are used do they comply
     with Part 8 ?   Yes ☐   No ☐

2.2.1.1 Suspension ropes (continued)

(i) If socketed anchors are used, state with which
British Standard they comply :   BS   N/A

(j) Are rope anchorages bound together ?   Yes [ ]   No [ ]

2.2.1.2 Suspension chains, state :   N/A [ ]

specified   actual

(1) Number

(2) The pitch

(3) The type and construction

(4) The relevant Standard

(5) Is the chain test certificate
available and in order ?   Yes [ ]   No [ ]

2.2.2 Safety gear   N/A [ ]

(a) Has the safety gear been certified as complying
with F.3 and in accordance with F.3.5. of Part 2 ?   Yes [ ]   No [ ]

(b) If foregoing answer is 'Yes' is the data plate fitted
and in accordance with 15.14 of Part 2 ?   Yes [ ]   No [ ]

(c) Is the safety gear sealed ?   Instantaneous   N/A [ ]   Yes [ ]   No [ ]

Progressive   N/A [ ]   Yes [ ]   No [ ]

2.2.3 Car

(a) State the internal width (wall to wall)
(without finishes) :

(b) State the internal depth (front return to rear wall or
front return to rear return) (without finishes) :

(c) Does the available internal floor area, related to
rated load and maximum number of passengers,
comply with 8.2 of Part 2 ?   Yes [ ]   No [ ]

2.2.4 Energy accumulation buffers (e.g. spring)

(a) If fitted, do buffers comply to 10.4.1. of Part 2 ?

N/A ☐

Yes ☐   No ☐

Note : It is recommended that buffers should have been identified with their spring rate maximum load and maker's name.

State quantity   Qty : ☐

State type if other than spring   Type : ☐

or

2.2.5 Energy dissipation buffers (e.g. oil)

N/A ☐

(a) Are they correctly filled and not leaking ?

Yes ☐   No ☐

(b) Is the stroke of each buffer in accordance with 10.4.3 of Part 2 ?

Yes ☐   No ☐

2.2.6 Hydraulic fluid (see BS 4231)

Maker : ☐   Type : ☐   Viscosity grade : ☐

2.2.7 Overspeed governor

N/A ☐

(a) Has the governor been certified as complying with F.4 and as being in accordance with F4.3 of Part 2 ?

Yes ☐   No ☐

(b) Is the data plate in accordance with 15.6 of Part 2 ?

Yes ☐   No ☐

(c) Is the governor sealed ?

Yes ☐   No ☐

2.2.8 Overspeed governor rope of safety rope

N/A ☐

(a) Is the nominal diameter of rope appropriate ?

Yes ☐   No ☐

specified   actual

State size : ☐ ☐

2.2.9 Landing doors and surrounds

N/A ☐

(a) Does the contract require that the landing doors and surrounds satisfy appropriate fire rating requirements ?

Yes ☐   No ☐

If so, what is the fire rating requirement ? ☐ h

(b) If the answer to (a) is Yes, is the test certificate available and in order ?

Yes ☐   No ☐

2.2.9 Landing doors and surrounds

(c) If so, and doors are manually operated, is the means of fire protection a fusible link ?

Yes ☐ No ☐

If the answer is 'No', describe method used : ☐

(d) Are the fire rated elements of the door assembly correctly fitted ?

Yes ☐ No ☐

2.2.10 Door locks

(a) Have the door locks been certified as complying with F.1.4 of Part 2 ?

Yes ☐ No ☐

If 'Yes' does the data plate comply with 15.13 of Part 2 ?

Yes ☐ No ☐

2.3 Static examination, electrical

2.3.1 Insulation resistance to earth (see clause 5)

(a) pump motor ☐ $M\Omega$ (b) power system ☐ $M\Omega$ (c) safety circuits ☐ $M\Omega$

2.3.2 Earthing

(a) Is the maximum continuity resistance to earth less than 0.5Ω ?

Yes ☐ No ☐

(b) Is the car connected to controller earthing terminal by a separate conductor no smaller than 0.75 mm^2 ?

Yes ☐ No ☐

(c) Does the earth loop impedance comply with fuse rating ?

Yes ☐ No ☐ reading ☐

2.3.3 Protection of conductors

(a) Is the fixed wiring in conduit (or trunking, or fittings which ensure equivalent protection throughout) ?

Yes ☐ No ☐

or

(b) If 'No' do cables comply with 13.5.1.2. of Part 2 ?

N/A ☐ Yes ☐ No ☐

2.3.4 Phase failure device

Does the phase reversal and phase failure protection operate correctly ?

Yes ☐ No ☐

2.3.5 Electrical conductors

Do the electrical conductors, including travelling cables, comply with 13.5.1 Part 2 ?

Yes ☐ No ☐

2.4 Dynamic tests

2.4.1 Safety contacts/circuits

(a) Have the contacts at each landing entrance been proved so that when open circuited there is no movement of the car outside the unlocking zone ?

Yes ☐ No ☐

2.4.1 Safety contacts/circuits

(b) Have the car door/gate contacts been proved so that when open circuited there is no car movement outside the unlocking zone ? Yes ☐ No ☐

(c) Have the stopping devices on car top and in the pulley room and pit been proved so that when open circuited no movement of the car occurs ? Yes ☐ No ☐

(d) Have all other switches/contacts in safety circuits been proved so that when open circuited no movement of the car occurs ? Yes ☐ No ☐

(e) Does the earthing of the most remote contact (lock or push button) operate a fuse or trip a circuit breaker without delay ? Yes ☐ No ☐

(f) Have the mechanical locks at each landing entrance been provided for positive locking ? Yes ☐ No ☐

(g) If separate terminal stopping switches are fitted, do they operate satisfactorily ? N/A ☐ Yes ☐ No ☐

(h) Do the final limit switches operate satisfactorily ? Yes ☐ No ☐

(i) Final limit switch settings. State distance to operate beyond finished floor level.

	specified	actual
Top	50 - 75 mm	
Bottom	50 - 75 mm	

2.4.2 Car top control station – with a load of 75 kg

(a) Speed up : ☐ m/s   (b) Speed down : ☐ m/s

(b) Does the design and operation of car top station comply with clause 14.2.1.3 of Part 2 ? Yes ☐ No ☐

2.4.3 Clearances and runbys

(a) Will the car and ram assembly (and counterweight, if fitted) clear all obstacles when driven at slow speed :

(1) With the car and rated load on to and fully compressing the car buffers ? Yes ☐ No ☐

(2) With the ram fully extended to the ram stop ? Yes ☐ No ☐

(b) What is the distance to the first striking points above the car with the ram fully extended to the ram stop ? ☐ mm

(c) Overtravel of car above top floor level ? ☐ mm

(d) Overtravel of car below bottom floor level ? ☐ mm

(e) Is there clearance under ram with car on fully compressed buffers ? Yes ☐ No ☐

State the dimension ☐ mm

2.4 Dynamic tests (continued)

(f) Is there clearance above the ram/pulley
assembly with fully extended ram ? N/A [ ] Yes [ ] No [ ]

State the dimension [ ] mm

(g) With the car in its fully raised position, i.e. ram fully
extended, is there a sufficient space to accommodate
the rectangular block 0.5 m x 0.6 m x 0.8 m above the Yes [ ] No [ ]
car specified in 5.7.1.1 (d) of Part 2 ?

If no, are reduced headroom notices displayed on car
top and machine room ? Yes [ ] No [ ]

(h) With the car on its fully compressed buffers is there a
sufficient space to accommodate the rectangular block
0.5 m x 0.6 m x 1.0 m below the car specified in 5.7.2.3 (a) Yes [ ] No [ ]
of Part 2 ?

If no, are reduced headroom notices displayed in pit and
machine rooms ? Yes [ ] No [ ]

NOTE : The clear distance between the bottom of the pit and the
lowest part of the guide shoes or rollers of safety gear blocks,
toeguards or parts of vertical sliding doors should be at least
0.1 m.

2.4.4 Entrance clearances

(a) Is the horizontal distance between the sill of the car and
the sill of all landing doors 35 mm or less ? Yes [ ] No [ ]
For each set of doors

(b) Is the running clearance between door panels, and
between panels and uprights, lintels or sills 6mm or less ? Yes [ ] No [ ]

(c) Has it been established that no recess or projection on
the face of the sliding door panels exceeds 3 mm ? Yes [ ] No [ ]

(d) Is the distance between the inner surface of the well and
the sill and framework of the car entrance or door Yes [ ] No [ ]
<= 0.15 m or 0.2 m if over a height not exceeding 0.5 m (see
5.4.3.2 of Part 2) ?

(e) If the answer to (d) is 'No', is the car door mechanically
locked when away from the unlocking zone in Yes [ ] No [ ]
accordance with 8.11.1 of Part 2 ?

2.4.5 Door tests

NOTE: Where appropriate the following tests should be carried out with car and landing doors coupled

(a) How are the doors operated ? manually [ ] if so, answer f,h,i,j,k,l

powered [ ] if so, answer all except l

(b) Is the measured maximum force to prevent
closing, at the mid-point of travel, 150 N or less ? Yes [ ] No [ ]

State the figure recorded : [ ] N

2.4.5 Door tests (continued)

(c) Is the measured kinetic energy 10 J or less ? Yes ☐ No ☐

State the figure recorded : ☐

(d) Do all the protective devices reverse the doors in accordance with 7.5.2.1.1. of Part 2 ? Includes all mechanical or electrical devices supplied. Yes ☐ No ☐

(e) If the protective device is made inoperative :

(1) Do the doors remain open ? Yes ☐ No ☐

(2) Do the doors close with a kinetic energy not exceeding 4 J ? N/A ☐ Yes ☐ No ☐

(f) Is the unlocking zone less than 0.2 m above and below landing levels (or 0.35 m in the case of simultaneously operated car and landing doors) ? Check length of retiring ramp and position of lock roller. Yes ☐ No ☐

(g) Do the landing doors have an automatic self-closing mechanism ? Yes ☐ No ☐

(h) Is each set of the landing doors capable of being unlocked from the outside with an emergency key ? Yes ☐ No ☐

If not, why ? ☐

(i) Does the door motor protection system function correctly ? Yes ☐ No ☐

Does the retiring actuator protection system function correctly ? N/A ☐ Yes ☐ No ☐

(j) Form of electrical protection provided for the door motor

D.C. circuit breaker	☐	Timing relay	☐
Three phase circuit breaker	☐	Thermistors	☐
Overloads in each phase	☐	Other (state)	Fuses

Form of electrical protection provided for the retiring actuator

D.C. circuit breaker	☐	Timing relay	☐
Three phase circuit breaker	☐	Thermistors	☐
Overloads in each phase	☐	Other (state)	Fuses

State the relevant characteristics : CCT (swing) ODT/CDT (powered)

Time to operate ☐ S

Run current ☐ A

(k) Can the car doors be manually opened within the unlocking zone with a force of less than 300 N with the power off ? Yes ☐ No ☐

(l) Does "car here" indicator comply with 7.6.2. of Part 2 for manual doors ? N/A ☐

2.5 Measurements of the hydraulic and electrical system

(1) With the car at highest floor level, state static
hydraulic pressure with :

Car empty	bar
Car with rated load	bar

(a) Provide the following details of the pump motor (as stated on data plate)

(1)	Maker :	
(2)	Serial No. :	
(3)	Type :	
(4)	AC voltage :	V
(5)	Power rating HP & kW :	HP kW
(6)	Current rating :	A
(7)	Speed :	r/min
(8)	Class of insulation :	

(b) Provide the following details of the pump (as stated on data plate) :

(1)	Maker :	
(2)	Serial No. :	
(3)	Type :	
(4)	Oil rate flow :	1/min

2.5 Measurements of the hydraulic and electrical system (continued)

(c) Measure and record the following operational data when the car is at mid point of travel :

Car loading condition		(see note 1) hydraulic pressure bar	lift speed m/s (see note 4)	lift motor input (see note 2)		levelling deviation +, - (see note 3) mm
				V	A	
empty	up					
	down					
half load	up					
	down					
rated	up					
	down					
rated + 10%	up					
	down					

NOTES :
1. The pressure readings should be taken between the check valve or down direction valve and the supply line to the cylinder.
2. The motor current readings should be measured on the main supply side of the line conductors of the motor within the control panel.
3. The maximum deviation should be stated in the appropriate box (i.e. one entry only).
4. Empty speed readings will be No Load + 1 person on top of the lift car.

(d) Pressure relief valve operated at pressure : [   ] bar

(e) High pressure switch set at [   ] bar

Low pressure switch set at N/A [   ] [   ] bar

(f) Is the presure relief valve secured against unauthorised interference ? Yes [   ] No [   ]

(g) Does the check valve hold the car with rated load at floor level ? Yes [   ] No [   ]

(h) Does the rupture valve function correctly ? Yes [   ] No [   ]

Distance travelled [   ] mm

(i) Does the resistor function correctly ? N/A [   ] Yes [   ] No [   ]

(j) Does the hand pump function correctly ? N/A [   ] Yes [   ] No [   ]

(k) Does the operation of the manual lowering valve lower the car at a speed not exceeding 0.3 m/s ? Yes [   ] No [   ]

(l) With the power switch off in the case of an indirect acting lift when the car is manually lowered onto a prop, does the ram stop, when a slack chain or slack rope condition occurs ? N/A [   ] Yes [   ] No [   ]

(m) In the case of an indirect acting lift, does the slack chain/rope switch or pressure switch prevent operation of the lift until pressure is re-established by re-setting the switch ? N/A [   ] Yes [   ] No [   ]

2.5 Measurements of the hydraulic and electrical system (continued)

(n) Are precautions against overheating the fluid provided ?   Yes ☐   No ☐

(o) Can the position of the lift car at any landing zone be detached from the lift motor room with the main power switched off ?   Yes ☐   No ☐

2.6 Pump motor main windings over current protective devices

(a) Measure and record the following (as appropriate) :

Type of device	Manual reset		Automatic reset		Time to operate		Trip current	
Three phase circuit breaker								
Overloads in each phase								
Timing relay (TR1)								
Thermistor (TCU)								
Other : name type								

(b) Have you found these to operate satisfactorily ?   Yes ☐   No ☐

2.7 Overspeed governor tests

2.7.1 Car overspeed governor test   N/A ☐

Complete the following :

Governor type : _____

Serial No. : _____

Device	Tripping speed		Does it operate effectively?	
	Marked	Measured (car down)	Yes	No
Electrical		m/s		
Mechanical	m/s	m/s		

2.7.1 Car overspeed governor test (continued)

State how the governor was tested on the installation

2.7.2 Counterweight overspeed governor test   N/A

Complete the following :

Governor type :

Serial No. :

Device	Tripping speed		Does it operate effectively?	
	Marked	Measured (car down)	Yes	No
Electrical		m/s		
Mechanical	m/s	m/s		

State how the governor was tested on the installation :

2.8   Car safety gear tests

NOTE : The following tests should be conducted with the car descending.

2.8.1 Test of devices for uncontrolled movement of car direct acting lifts

N/A ☐

Combination	Selection 1	Selection 2	Selection 3	Selection 4
Free fall or descent with excessive speed				
Instantaneous safety gear/clamping device operated by overspeed governor	☐			
Progressive safety gear/clamping device operated by overspeed governor		☐		
Rupture valve			☐ ☐	
Restrictor				☐
		and		
Precautions against creeping				
Tripping of safety gear	☐	☐	☐ ☐	☐
or Clamping device	or	or	or	or
or PAWL device	☐	☐	☐ ☐	☐
	or	or	or	
or Electrical anti-creep	☐	☐	☐ ☐	

Indicate which selection combination to be tested

2.8.2 Test of devices for uncontrolled movement of the car, indirecting acting lifts

N/A ☐

Combination	Selection 1	2	Selection 3	4	Selection 5	6	Selection 7	8
Free fall or descent with excessive speed								
Instantaneous safety gear/clamping device operated by overspeed governor	☐							
Progressive wedge safety gear operated by overspeed governor		☐						
Instantaneous safety gear operated by suspension failure			☐					
Progressive wedge safety gear operated by suspension failure				☐				
Instantaneous safety gear operated by safety rope			and	and	☐		☐	
Progressive wedge safety gear operated by safety rope					and	☐ and	and	☐ and
Rupture valve			☐	☐	☐	☐		
Restrictor					and		☐	☐
Precautions against creeping								
Tripping of safety gear	☐	☐						
	or	or						
or PAWL device	☐	☐	☐	☐	☐	☐	☐	☐
	or	or	or	or	or	or		
or Electrical anti-creep	☐	☐	☐	☐	☐	☐	☐	☐

Indicate which selection combination to be tested

2.8.3 Safety gear tests with non-conventional car loading and oversize cars

N/A ☐

Is the design of the car, car sling, suspension, safety gear, rupture valve, clamping device, PAWL device, guide rails and buffers based on a load resulting from Table 1.1 ?

Yes ☐   No ☐

2.8.4 Test

(a) To carry out the safety gear tests, the test load must be uniformly distributed in the car. The safety gear switch, overspeed governor switch, buffer switch or any other electrical devices that may cause the lift to stop by hydraulic means must be temporarily sorted out.

N/A ☐

(b) Does the stopping device operate correctly ?

Yes ☐   No ☐

(c) For progressive safety gear state slide distance :

☐ mm

(d) Is the floor horizontal or sloping less than 5% (1 in 11) ?

Yes ☐   No ☐

NOTES :

1. Test speeds
   (a) Use rated speed for all safety gear clamping and PAWL devices
   (b) Rupture valve : According to data plate
   (c) Restrictor : Maximum speed not to exceed down speed + 0.3 m/s

2. Test loads
   (a) Conventional car loading to table 1.1 clause 8.2.1. of Part 2
       i. Use rated load for instantaneous safety gears, rupture valves and restrictors
       ii. Use 125% of rated load for progressive safety gears, clamping devices, PAWL devices and instantaneous safety gear with buffered effect
   (b) Non-conventional car loading to table 1.1.A clause 8.2.2. of Part 2
       i. Use 125% of rated load for instantaneous safety gears with buffered effect, clamping devices and PAWL devices
       ii. Use 150% of rated load for progressive safety gears
       iii Use rated load for rupture valves and restrictors

2.8.5. Counterweight and rope safety gear

N/A ☐

(a) Counterweight safety gear :

Yes ☐   No ☐

   Test load = empty car

   Test speed = car up rated speed

(b) For progressive safety gear state slide distance :

☐ m

(c) Does this value fall within those given in appendix ?

Yes ☐   No ☐

2.8.6. Safety rope

(a) If the safety gear is tripped by a safety rope
does the triggering mechanism operate satisfactorily ?   N/A ☐   Yes ☐   No ☐

(b) Does the slack rope safety switch function
correctly ?   N/A ☐   Yes ☐   No ☐

(c) State rope size :   See 2.2.8. (a)   ☐ mm

2.9 Hydraulic system pressure test

(a) When subjected to 200% of the pressure applied
between the non-return valve and the jack (included) for a
period of 5 minutes, is pressure maintained with no
evidence of hydraulic fluid leakage ?   Yes ☐   No ☐

(b) Pressure relief valve operates at pressure.   ☐ bar See 2.5. (e) & (g)

(c) Is pressure relief valve secured against unauthorized
interference ?   Yes ☐   No ☐

NOTE : This test must be carried out after tests for precautions against free fall or descent with excessive speeds

2.10 Buffers

2.10.1 Energy dissipation type (e.g. oil)   N/A ☐

(a) For car buffers, when the car was brought into contact
with the buffers at the rated load, at rated speed or at a speed
for which the stroke of the buffers has been calculated, was
operation satisfactory ?   Yes ☐   No ☐

(b) For counterweight buffers, when the counterweight
was brought into contact with the buffer with the car empty at
rated speed, or at a speed for which the stroke of the buffer
has been calculated, was the operation satisfactory ?   Yes ☐   No ☐

(c) Do the buffers recover automatically after operation ?   Yes ☐   No ☐

or

2.10.2 Energy accumulation buffers (e.g. spring)   N/A ☐

NOTE : If answer to 2.2.4. (a) in this sample certificate is "Yes" no test required.

2.11 Anti-creep

(a) Does the device only operate within the door unlocking zone ?   Yes ☐   No ☐

(b) Does the device start to operate within a maximum of 120 mm below floor
level but within the door unlocking zone ?   Yes ☐   No ☐

2.11 Anti-creep (continued)

(c) Does the device operate with the car and landing doors both open and closed ?   Yes ☐   No ☐

(d) Is the isolating switch in the machine room marked with the legend "Switch to be kept closed at all times except during maintenance and repair" ?   Yes ☐   No ☐

(e) Does the device comply with Table 2 of 9.5 of Part 2 ?   Yes ☐   No ☐

(f) Does car top control and pit switch isolate relevelling ?   Yes ☐   No ☐

2.12 Duty cycle test

(a) Does the lift operate satisfactorily for a period of at least 0.5 hours when running with rated load, full travel and intermediate stops at a rate of starts at least equal to the number of starts recommended in Part 6 ?   Yes ☐   No ☐

(b) If answer is "No" state reasons :

NOTE : It may be necessary to reduce open timing to achieve the required number of starts per hour

2.13 General

(a) Is the maximum load indicated in the car (e.g. number of persons, kg and identification no.) and does it comply with 15.2.1 of Part 2 ?   Yes ☐   No ☐

(b) Does the fire-fighting control system comply with the recommendations given in BS 5588 : Part 5 ?   N/A ☐   Yes ☐   No ☐

(c) Does the disabled evacuation system comply with the recommendations given in BS 5588 : Part 5 ?   N/A ☐   Yes ☐   No ☐

(d) Are the emergency instructions displayed in the machine room ?   Yes ☐   No ☐

(e) Does the emergency operation system(s) function correctly in accordance with 12.5 of Part 1 ?   Yes ☐   No ☐

If 'Yes', to whom has it been demonstrated ?

Name :

Organisation :

2.13. General (continued)

(f) Is the machine room artificial lighting adequate
for maintenance purposes ?   Yes ☐   No ☐

(g) Does the artificial lighting in the well comply with
5.9. of Part 2 ?   Yes ☐   No ☐

(h) Are the machine room conditions satisfactory ?   Yes ☐   No ☐

If the answer is 'No', state reasons : _____

(i) Is the machine room adequately ventilated ?   Yes ☐   No ☐

(j) State the machine room temperature at the end
of tests :   _____

Is the temperature rise acceptable ?   Yes ☐   No ☐

(k) Are the machine room doors or trap doors fitted
with a suitable lock complying with 6.3.3.3. of Part 2 ?   Yes ☐   No ☐

(l) What are the means of emergency
communication for passengers in the lift car ?   _____

Do they work ?   Yes ☐   No ☐

(m) Does the emergency lighting of the car stay
illuminated for one hour ?   Yes ☐   No ☐

If the answer is 'No', state reasons : _____

(o) Are the safety notices/instructions specified in
clause 15 of Part 1 and recommended in Part 6 correctly
displayed ?   Yes ☐   No ☐

(p) Has a car apron been fitted ?   Yes ☐   No ☐

(q) Has a counterweight screen been fitted ?   N/A ☐

2.14 Conclusions

(a) Is the lift installation complete and ready to be put into service ?   Yes [ ]   No [ ]

Note : Some items requring attention may not be part of the contract for the lift
but part of the installation and the responsibility of others. A list of inclusions
and exclusions is given in Part 6

(b) If the answer to (a) is 'No', provide details in space below :

[   ]

2.15 Declaration

I/We certify that on [   ] the equipment was thoroughly examined and found to be free from obvious
defects and to comply with British Standard BS 5655 : Part 2, subject to any statement in 2.1.4 (b) above
and that the foregoing is a correct report of the result.

Signature (s) :   [   ]   [   ]

Name and address of public service, association, company, firm or person making the examination :

[   ]   [   ]

Position in above organisation of the person who conducted the examination :

[   ]   [   ]

or

Qualifications of examiner, if working on his own account :

[   ]   [   ]

References

Acts and Regulations

The Building Act 1984. HMSO 1984.

Disabled Persons Act 1981. HMSO 1981.

Disabled Persons (Northern Ireland) Act. HMSO 1989.

Factories Act 1961. HMSO 1961.

Fire Precautions Act 1971. HMSO 1971.

Fire Safety and Safety of Places of Sport Act 1987. HMSO 1987.

Health and Safety at Work etc Act 1974. HMSO 1974.

SI 3140:1994 The Construction (Design and Management) Regulations. HMSO 1994.

SI 635:1989 Electricity at Work Regulations. HMSO 1989.

SI 13:1991 Electricity at Work Regulations (Northern Ireland). HMSO 1991.

SI 2372:1992 The Electromagnetic Compatibility Regulations. HMSO 1992.

SI 3021:1994 The Electromagnetic Compatibility (Amendment) Regulations. HMSO 1994.

SI 1821:1984 (NI 11) Fire Services (Northern Ireland) Order. HMSO 1984.

SR 404:1993 Fire Services (1984 Order) (Modifications) (Northern Ireland) Regulations. HMSO 1993.

SI 1380:1990 Health and Safety (Training for Employment) Regulations. HMSO 1990.

SI 1:1994 Health and Safety (Training for Employment) Regulations (Northern Ireland). HMSO 1994.

SI 1039:1978 (NI 9) Health and Safety at Work (Northern Ireland) Order. HMSO 1978.

SI 195:1992 Lifting Plant and Equipment (Record of Test and Examination etc) Regulations. HMSO 1992.

SR 366:1993 Lifting Plant and Equipment (Record of Test and Examination etc) Regulations (Northern Ireland). HMSO 1993.

SI 2051:1992 The Management of Health and Safety at Work Regulations. HMSO 1992.

SI 459:1992 The Management of Health and Safety at Work Regulations (Northern Ireland). HMSO 1992.

SI 849:1968 Offices, Shops and Railway Premises (Hoists and Lifts) Regulations. HMSO 1968.

SR 26:1969 Office and Shop Premises (Hoists and Lifts) Regulations (Northern Ireland). HMSO 1969.

SI 2023:1985 Reporting of Injuries, Diseases and Dangerous Occurrences Regulations. HMSO 1985.

SR 247:1986 Reporting of Injuries, Diseases and Dangerous Occurrences Regulations (Northern Ireland). HMSO 1986.

SI 3073:1992 The Supply of Machinery (Safety) Regulations. HMSO 1992.

SI 2063:1994 The Supply of Machinery (Safety) (Amendment) Regulations. HMSO 1994.

SI 3004:1992 The Workplace (Health, Safety and Welfare) Regulations. HMSO 1992.

SR 37:1993 The Workplace (Health, Safety and Welfare) Regulations (Northern Ireland). HMSO 1993.

Building Regulations and related publications

SI 2768:1991 The Building Regulations. HMSO 1991.

SI 1180:1992 The Building Regulations (Amendment) Regulations. HMSO 1992.

SI 2179:1990 (S 187) The Building Standards (Scotland) Regulations. HMSO 1990.

SR 243:1994 Building Regulations (Northern Ireland). HMSO 1994.

The Building Regulations 1991: approved documents A–N. Department of the Environment, HMSO 1992.

The Building Regulations 1991: approved document to support regulation 7. Department of the Environment, HMSO 1992.

The Building Regulations (Northern Ireland) 1994 – Technical booklets C–E, G1, H, P, R and V. Department of the Environment for Northern Ireland, HMSO 1994.

The Building Standards (Scotland) Regulations 1990: Technical standards. Scottish Office Building Directorate, HMSO 1990.

NHS Estates and Scottish Office publications

National Health Service Model Engineering Specifications (Electrical vol. 1)

   Electric traction lifts (C42A). NHS Estates, 1993.

   Hydraulic lifts (C42B). NHS Estates, 1993.

   Service lifts (C42C). NHS Estates, 1993.

Health Building Note 40 – Common activity spaces

   Volume 4: Circulation areas. NHS Estates, HMSO 1995.

SHPN 1 – Health service building in Scotland. Scottish Office, HMSO 1991.

SHPN 2 – Hospital briefing and operational policies. Scottish Office, HMSO 1993.

Health Technical Memoranda (HTMs)

HTM 2007 – Electrical services: supply and distribution. HMSO 1993.

HTM 2011 – Emergency electrical services. HMSO 1993.

HTM 2014 – Abatement of electrical interference. HMSO 1993.

HTM 2020 – Electrical safety code for low voltage systems (Escode – LV). HMSO 1993.

HTM 2021 – Electrical safety code for high voltage systems (Escode – HV). HMSO 1994.

HTM 2050 – Risk management in the NHS estate. HMSO 1994.

Firecode publications

Firecode: policy and principles. NHS Estates, HMSO 1994.

Firecode: Nucleus fire precautions recommendations. Department of Health, HMSO 1989.

HTM 81 – Fire precautions in new hospitals. DHSS, HMSO 1987. (new edition in preparation)

HTM 81 Supplement 1 – Fire precautions in new hospitals. NHS Estates, HMSO 1993.

HTM 83 – Fire safety in healthcare premises: general fire precautions. NHS Estates, HMSO 1994.

HTM 85 – Fire precautions in existing hospitals. NHS Estates, HMSO 1994.

HTM 86 – Fire risk assessment in hospitals. NHS Estates, HMSO 1994.

Fire Practice Note 3 – Escape bed lifts. Department of Health, HMSO 1987.

Firecode in Scotland: policy and principles. Scottish Office Home and Health Department, HMSO 1994.

Fire safety: new health buildings in Scotland. Scottish Home and Health Department, HMSO 1987.

British Standards

BS4737 Intruder alarm systems.

   Part 1:1986   **Specification for installed systems with local audible and/or remote signalling.**
             (AMD 5804, 12/87)

BS5588 Fire precautions in the design, construction and use of buildings.

   Part 3:1991   **Code of practice for office buildings.**

   Part 5:1991   **Code of practice for fire-fighting stairs and lifts.**
             (AMD 7196, 6/92)

   Part 8:1988   **Code of practice for means of escape for disabled people.**

BS5655 Lifts and service lifts

   Part 1:1986   **Safety rules for the construction and installation of electric lifts (implementing EN 81:Part 1). To be used in conjunction with PD 6500:1986 Explanatory supplement to BS5655:Part 1.**
             (AMD 5840, 9/89)

Part 2:1988 Safety rules for the construction and installation of hydraulic lifts (implementing EN 81:Part 2). *(AMD 6220, 4/89)*

Part 3:1989 Specification for electric service lifts. *(AMD 6377, 9/91)*

Part 5:1989 Specification for dimensions of standard lift arrangements.

Part 6:1990 Code of practice for selection and installation.

Part 7:1983 Specification for manual control devices, indicators and additional fittings (implementing ISO 4190–5). *(AMD 4912, 9/85)*

Part 8:1983 Specification for eyebolts for lift suspension.

Part 9:1985 Specification for guide rails. *(AMD 5186, 7/86; AMD 5786, 1/88)*

Part 10:1986 Specification for testing and inspection of electric and hydraulic lifts. *(AMD 6002, 5/89)*

Part 11:1989 Recommendation for the installation of new, and the modernisation of, electric lifts in existing buildings. *(AMD 8097, 3/94)*

Part 12:1989 Recommendation for the installation of new, and the modernisation of, hydraulic lifts in existing buildings. *(AMD 6762, 9/91; AMD 8098, 3/94)*

BS5810:1979 Code of practice for access for the disabled to buildings.

BS7255:1989 Code of practice for safe working on lifts *(AMD 6375, 4/91)*

BS EN ISO 9000 Quality management and quality assurance standards

Health and Safety Executive publications

Lifts: thorough examination and testing (PM 7). Health and Safety Executive, HMSO 1982.

Safety at lift landings (PM 26). Health and Safety Executive, HMSO 1981.

Lifting Plant and Equipment (Records of Test and Examination etc) Regulations 1992. Record of thorough examination of lifting plant equipment (Form F2530). Health and Safety Executive, HMSO. (issued in pads of 10)

Miscellaneous publications

CIBSE Commissioning codes

Series A: Air distribution systems. Chartered Institute of Building Services Engineers (CIBSE) 1971.

Series D: Transportation systems in buildings. Chartered Institute of Building Services Engineers (CIBSE) 1993.

National Association of Lift Makers (NALM) Distance Learning Course, Course Reference Books

Other publications in this series

(Given below are details of all Health Technical Memoranda available from HMSO. HTMs marked (*) are currently being revised, those marked (†) are out of print. Some HTMs in preparation at the time of publication of this HTM are also listed.)

1   Anti-static precautions: rubber, plastics and fabrics†

2   Anti-static precautions: flooring in anaesthetising areas (and data processing rooms), 1977.

3   –

4   –

5   Steam boiler plant instrumentation†

6   Protection of condensate systems: filming amines†

2007 Electrical services: supply and distribution, 1993.

8   –

2009 Pneumatic tube transport systems, 1995.

2010 Sterilizers, 1994, 1995.

2011 Emergency electrical services, 1993.

12   –

13   –

2014 Abatement of electrical interference, 1993.

2015 Bedhead services, 1994.

16   –

17   Health building engineering installations: commissioning and associated activities, 1978.

18   Facsimile telegraphy: possible applications in DGHs†

19   Facsimile telegraphy: the transmission of pathology reports within a hospital – a case study†

2020 Electrical safety code for low voltage systems, 1993.

2021 Electrical safety code for high voltage systems, 1993.

2022 Medical gas pipeline systems, 1994.

2023 Access and accommodation for engineering services, 1995.

2025 Ventilation in healthcare premises, 1994.

26   Commissioning of oil, gas and dual fired boilers: with notes on design, operation and maintenance†

2027 Hot and cold water supply, storage and mains services, 1995.

28 to 29 –

2030 Washer-disinfectors

31 to 39 –

2040 The control of legionellae in healthcare premises – a code of practice, 1993.

41 to 49 –

2050 Risk assessment in the NHS estate, 1994.

51 to 53 –

2055 Telecommunications (telephone exchanges), 1994.

Component Data Base (HTMs 54 to 80)

54.1 User manual, 1993.

55   Windows, 1989.

56   Partitions, 1989.

57   Internal glazing, 1995.

58   Internal doorsets, 1989.

59   Ironmongery†

60   Ceilings, 1989.

61   Flooring, 1995.

62   Demountable storage systems, 1989.

63   Fitting storage systems, 1989.

64   Sanitary assemblies, 1995.

65   Health signs*

66   Cubicle curtain track, 1989.

67   Laboratory fitting-out system, 1993.

68   Ducts and panel assemblies, 1993.

69   Protection, 1993.

70   Fixings, 1993.

71   Materials management modular storage system*

72 to 80 –

Firecode

81   Firecode: fire precautions in new hospitals*

81   Supp 1, 1993.

82   Firecode: alarm and detection systems, 1989.

83   Fire safety in healthcare premises: general fire precautions, 1994.

85   Firecode: fire precautions in existing hospitals, 1994.

86   Firecode: fire risk assessment in hospitals, 1994.

87   Firecode: textiles and furniture, 1993.

88   Fire safety in health care premises: guide to fire precautions in NHS housing in the community for mentally handicapped/ill people, 1986.

New HTMs in preparation

2035 Mains signalling

2005 Building management systems

2045 Acoustics

2031 Steam supply for sterilizers

Health Technical Memoranda published by HMSO can be purchased from HMSO bookshops in London (post orders to PO Box 276, SW8 5DT), Edinburgh, Belfast, Manchester, Birmingham and Bristol, or through good booksellers. HMSO provide a copy service for publications which are out of print; and a standing order service.

Enquiries about Health Technical Memoranda (but not orders) should be addressed to: NHS Estates, Department of Health, 1 Trevelyan Square, Boar Lane, Leeds LS1 6AE.

About NHS Estates

NHS Estates is an Executive Agency of the Department of Health and is involved with all aspects of health estate management, development and maintenance. The Agency has a dynamic fund of knowledge which it has acquired during 30 years of working in the field. Using this knowledge NHS Estates has developed products which are unique in range and depth. These are described below. NHS Estates also makes its experience available to the field through its consultancy services.

Enquiries about NHS Estates should be addressed to:
NHS Estates, Department of Health,
1 Trevelyan Square, Boar Lane, Leeds LS1 6AE.
Telephone 0113 254 7000.

Some other NHS Estates products

Activity Database – a computerised system for defining the activities which have to be accommodated in spaces within the health buildings. *NHS Estates*

Estatecode – user manual for managing a health estate. Includes a recommended methodology for property appraisal and provides a basis for integration of the estate into corporate business planning. *HMSO*

Concode – outlines proven methods of selecting contracts and commissioning consultants. Reflects official policy on contract procedures. *HMSO*

Works Information Management System – a computerised information system for estate management tasks, enabling tangible assets to be put into the context of servicing requirements. *NHS Estates*

Health Building Notes – advice for project teams procuring new buildings and adapting or extending existing buildings. *HMSO*

Health Guidance Notes – an occasional series of publications which respond to changes in Department of Health policy or reflect changing NHS operational management. Each deals with a specific topic and is complementary to a related HTM. *HMSO*

Health Facilities Notes – debate current and topical issues of concern across all areas of healthcare provision. *HMSO*

Firecode – for policy, technical guidance and specialist aspects of fire precautions. *HMSO*

Capital Investment Manual Database – software support for managing the capital programme. Compatible with the Capital Investment Manual. *NHS Estates*

Model Engineering Specifications – comprehensive advice used in briefing consultants, contractors and suppliers of healthcare engineering services to meet Departmental policy and best practice guidance. *NHS Estates*

Quarterly Briefing – gives a regular overview on the construction industry and an outlook on how this may affect building projects in the health sector, in particular the impact on business prices. Also provides information on new and revised cost allowances for health buildings. Published four times a year; available on subscription direct from NHS Estates. *NHS Estates*

Works Guidance Index – an annual, fully cross-referenced index listing all NHS Estates publications and other documents related to the construction and equipping of health buildings. *NHS Estates*

Items noted "HMSO" can be purchased from HMSO Bookshops in London (post orders to PO Box 276, SW8 5DT), Edinburgh, Belfast, Manchester, Birmingham and Bristol or through good booksellers.

NHS Estates consultancy services

Designed to meet a range of needs from advice on the oversight of estates management functions to a much fuller collaboration for particularly innovative or exemplary projects.

Enquiries should be addressed to: NHS Estates Consultancy Service (address as above).

Printed in the United Kingdom for HMSO
Dd 0300494 C14 9/95 9385 2409

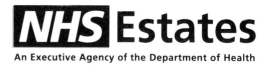

An Executive Agency of the Department of Health

Department of Health
1 Trevelyan Square
Boar Lane
Leeds
LS1 6AE
Fax 0113 254 7299
Telephone 0113 254 7000

Dear Customer

OLD

At NHS Estates, we constantly strive to produce publications that are relevant to the demands of the NHS and our worldwide healthcare customers.

It would help us to provide you with a better service if you could set aside a few minutes to complete the questionnaire on the reverse, fold as shown and return in a window envelope.

Win a free Health Building Note of your choice.

As a token of appreciation for taking the time to complete this card, all cards will be placed into an annual draw. The winning entry will receive a free Health Building Note of their choice.

Thank you for your comments.

John Locke
Chief Executive

There are no cash alternatives to the prize offered.

OLD

- -

**JOHN LOCKE
CHIEF EXECUTIVE
NHS ESTATES
FREEPOST LS 5588
LEEDS
LS1 1YY**

September 1995 – HTM 2024 – Lifts – VALVER

Publication title .... Date ....

Reader Details

Name ....

Position ....

Organisation ....

Address ....

.... Postcode ....

Telephone ....

Please tick the appropriate box

	Very Good	Good	Fair	Poor
Appropriateness of subject	❑	❑	❑	❑
Met my need	❑	❑	❑	❑
Clarity of presentation	❑	❑	❑	❑
Quality of content	❑	❑	❑	❑
Value for money	❑	❑	❑	❑
Overall rating of the publication	❑	❑	❑	❑

Will you be purchasing further editions in the series?   YES ❑   NO ❑

Other comments / areas for improvement?

....

....

Do you have any suggested subjects for the future?

....

....

Do you receive copies of our quarterly Newslink Newsletter?   YES ❑   NO ❑

Do you wish to receive a copy?   YES ❑   NO ❑

Have you purchased other products / services from us recently?

Please tick

Other publications	❑	**Activity DataBase**	❑
Consultancy services	❑	**Wims Software Enhancements**	❑
Other software products	❑	**Other: Please specify**	❑

Are there any other ways NHS Estates can assist you?

....

....

....

How did you receive your copy?

Sent/Issued by NHSE ❑   **Purchased from HMSO** ❑